SMOOTHIES FOR WEIGHT LOSS

**Blend The Pounds Away With These
100 Delicious Recipes And Transform
Your Body With Nutrient-Packed
Blends Ready In 5 Minutes.**

"Sip To Shed"

**BY
AURORA HENDRIX**

Table Of Contents

Monthly Transformation Tracker: Your Personal Growth Compass!

Conclusion: Your Journey to a Healthier You
THANK YOU

Introduction

The Power of Smoothies for Weight Loss:

Smoothies have emerged as nutritional powerhouses, offering a delicious and convenient way to fuel our bodies. The quest for weight loss often involves navigating through complex diet plans and restrictive meal options. Enter the transformative world of smoothies – a simple yet effective solution that brings together taste and nutrition in a single glass.

The inherent power of smoothies for weight loss lies in their ability to combine essential nutrients, fiber, and hydration. When carefully crafted, these blends can be rich in vitamins, minerals, and antioxidants, providing a comprehensive approach to health and wellness. Unlike traditional dieting, where meals might feel like a sacrifice, smoothies offer a delightful and satisfying experience. They become a lifestyle choice rather than a temporary fix.

A key aspect of smoothies is their versatility. Whether you're a fan of green vegetables, fruits, or protein-packed ingredients, there's a smoothie recipe tailored to your preferences. The amalgamation of diverse ingredients allows for a broad spectrum of nutrients, contributing to a balanced and sustainable weight loss journey. Moreover, the ease of customization makes smoothies accessible to individuals with various dietary requirements.

Beyond the nutritional benefits, the liquid form of smoothies ensures efficient nutrient absorption. The blending process breaks down fruits, vegetables, and other components into a more easily digestible state, promoting quicker absorption and utilization by the body. This aids in sustained energy levels, keeping you fueled throughout the day.

Why "Sip To Shed"?

"Sip To Shed" encapsulates the essence of our journey towards weight loss through smoothies. It's not just a catchy phrase but a philosophy that embodies the simplicity and effectiveness of incorporating smoothies into our daily routine.

Sipping implies a gradual and enjoyable process, echoing the idea that weight loss doesn't have to be an arduous task. By sipping on nutrient-packed blends, we shift the focus from rigid dieting to a more holistic and sustainable approach. The act of sipping also encourages mindfulness, fostering a connection with what we consume and promoting healthier eating habits.

"Shed" signifies the shedding of excess weight, both physically and metaphorically. The journey to shed pounds is not just about numbers on a scale but about shedding unhealthy habits, negative mindsets, and embracing a positive change. **"Sip To Shed"** encourages a gradual, consistent transformation rather than quick fixes.

This phrase serves as a daily reminder that each sip is a step towards a healthier, lighter version of ourselves. It's an invitation to embark on a journey where weight loss becomes a natural byproduct of nourishing our bodies with wholesome ingredients. **"Sip To Shed"** is not just a tagline; it's an empowering mantra that guides us through a delicious and rewarding path to a better, more vibrant life.

GETTING STARTED:

Embarking on a smoothie journey for weight loss requires a well-stocked arsenal of ingredients and a few key tools. These essentials lay the foundation for creating nutrient-dense and satisfying blends that contribute to your health goals.

Ingredients:

1. Leafy Greens: Spinach, kale, and Swiss chard add a nutrient-packed punch without overwhelming the taste.
2. Fruits: Berries, bananas, and citrus fruits bring sweetness, fiber, and a variety of vitamins.
3. Protein Sources: Greek yogurt, almond butter, or protein powder contribute to a filling and muscle-nourishing smoothie.

4. Liquid Base: Almond milk, coconut water, or plain water provide hydration and help achieve the desired consistency.

5. Healthy Fats: Avocado, chia seeds, or flaxseeds offer essential fats for satiety and overall well-being.

6. Superfoods: Additions like spirulina, matcha, or acai berries bring an extra boost of antioxidants and nutrients.

Tools:

1. High-Quality Blender: Invest in a powerful blender to ensure a smooth and creamy texture, breaking down tough ingredients for optimal nutrient absorption.

2. Measuring Cups and Spoons: Accurate measurements help maintain the nutritional balance of your smoothies.

3. Storage Containers: Prepare ingredients in advance and store them in labeled containers for quick and easy assembly.

4. Strainer: For those who prefer a smoother texture, a strainer can help remove pulp and seeds.

5. Reusable Straws: Make sipping your smoothie an eco-friendly experience while also enhancing the overall enjoyment.

Tips for Effective Weight Loss with Smoothies:

Creating weight-loss-friendly smoothies involves more than just throwing ingredients into a blender. These tips ensure that your smoothie journey is not only delicious but also effective in achieving your health and fitness goals.

Balance Macronutrients:

Ensure a balanced blend of carbohydrates, proteins, and healthy fats in each smoothie. This combination provides sustained energy, keeps you full, and supports muscle health.

Watch Portion Sizes:

While smoothies are nutritious, it's crucial to be mindful of portion sizes to control calorie intake. Use measuring tools until you become familiar with appropriate amounts.

Prioritize Whole Ingredients:

Opt for whole, unprocessed ingredients to maximize nutritional benefits. Fresh fruits, vegetables, and minimally processed additives contribute to overall well-being.

Control Added Sugars:

Be cautious with sweeteners and avoid excessive added sugars. Rely on the natural sweetness of fruits and consider using alternatives like honey or maple syrup in moderation.

Experiment with Greens:

If you're new to incorporating greens into your smoothies, start with milder options like spinach. Gradually experiment with kale and other leafy greens to find what suits your taste buds.

Hydration Matters:

Use hydrating bases like coconut water or plain water to boost hydration. Staying well-hydrated supports overall health and complements the weight loss process.

Include Protein:

Protein is a key player in weight loss, promoting a feeling of fullness and supporting muscle maintenance. Incorporate sources like Greek yogurt, protein powder, or nut butter.

Pre-Prep Ingredients:

Streamline your routine by prepping ingredients in advance. Wash, chop, and store fruits and
vegetables, so they're readily available when you're ready to blend. This not only saves time but also encourages consistency in your smoothie-making routine.

Mindful Blending:

Take the time to blend your ingredients thoroughly. This ensures a smooth consistency and maximizes the absorption of nutrients. Blend leafy greens and harder ingredients first bcforc adding liquids and softer elements.

Incorporate Fiber:

Fiber is a secret weapon for weight loss as it aids digestion and promotes a feeling of fullness. Keep the fiber content high by including fruits with skins, seeds, or adding a tablespoon of flaxseeds.

Temperature Matters:

If you prefer a chilled smoothie, consider using frozen fruits or adding ice cubes. The cool temperature can enhance the refreshing experience and may even slightly boost metabolism.

Customize According to Your Goals:

Tailor your smoothies to match your specific weight loss and fitness goals. Adjust ingredient quantities, types, and ratios based on your individual needs and preferences.

Enjoy Variety:

Keep your smoothie routine exciting by incorporating a variety of ingredients. This not only ensures a diverse range of nutrients but also prevents taste fatigue, making it more likely that you'll stick to your healthy habits.

Listen to Your Body:

Pay attention to how your body responds to different ingredients. Some may find certain combinations more satiating or energizing, while others might need adjustments based on their digestive sensitivities.

Monitor Total Caloric Intake:
While smoothies can be a fantastic addition to a weight loss plan, they should be part of a well-rounded diet. Be mindful of your overall caloric intake and ensure that your smoothies complement, rather than replace, other essential nutrients.

Post-Workout Refuel:
Utilize smoothies as a post-workout refueling option. Including protein-rich ingredients can aid muscle recovery, especially after intense physical activity.

Keep Hydration Separate:
While smoothies contribute to your daily fluid intake, it's important to continue hydrating with plain water throughout the day. This maintains optimal hydration levels for overall health and wellness.

Incorporating these tips into your smoothie-making routine will not only enhance the weight loss benefits but also make the entire process more enjoyable and sustainable. Remember, the journey towards a healthier you is about progress, not perfection, and each nutrient-packed sip brings you closer to your wellness goals.

BREAKFAST BLENDS:

Energizing Morning Mix

Ingredients:
- ½ cup spinach
- ½ banana, frozen
- ½ cup blueberries
- ½ cup Greek yogurt
- ½ tablespoon chia seeds
- ½ cup almond milk

Instructions:
Blend spinach, frozen banana, blueberries, Greek yogurt, chia seeds, and almond milk until smooth. Enjoy the refreshing green energy to kickstart your day.

Berry Boost Breakfast

Ingredients:
- ½ cup mixed berries (strawberries, raspberries, and blackberries)
- ½ cup oats

- ½ cup plain yogurt
- ½ tablespoon honey
- ½ cup coconut water

Instructions:

Combine mixed berries, oats, yogurt, honey, and coconut water in a blender. Blend until creamy, providing a delightful berry-filled boost for a nutritious breakfast.

Green Goodness Wake-Up

Ingredients:
- ½ cup kale, stems removed
- ½ green apple, cored
- ½ cucumber, peeled
- ½ lemon, juiced
- ½ tablespoon ginger, grated
- ½ cup water or coconut water

Instructions:

Blend kale, green apple, cucumber, lemon juice, ginger, and water or coconut water until you achieve a vibrant green concoction. This green goodness is a refreshing and nutritious way to wake up your senses in the morning.

Tropical Sunrise Delight

Ingredients:
- ½ cup pineapple chunks
- ½ cup mango, diced
- ½ orange, peeled
- ½ cup coconut milk
- ½ tablespoon flaxseeds
- ½ cup water or orange juice

Instructions:
Blend pineapple, mango, orange, coconut milk, flaxseeds, and water or orange juice until smooth. Experience a taste of the tropics to brighten your morning.

Peanut Butter Protein Punch

Ingredients:
- ½ banana, frozen
- ½ cup strawberries, hulled
- ½ cup milk (dairy or plant-based)
- ½ cup plain Greek yogurt
- ½ tablespoon peanut butter
- ½ teaspoon cinnamon

Instructions:

Blend frozen banana, strawberries, milk, Greek yogurt, peanut butter, and cinnamon for a protein-packed and satisfying breakfast punch.

Apple Cinnamon Oat Delight

Ingredients:
- ½ apple, cored and sliced
- ½ cup oats
- ½ cup almond milk
- ½ teaspoon cinnamon
- ½ tablespoon honey
- ½ cup ice cubes

Instructions:
Blend apple slices, oats, almond milk, cinnamon, honey, and ice cubes until creamy. Enjoy the comforting flavors of apple cinnamon goodness.

Citrus Zest Fusion

Ingredients:
- ½ orange, peeled
- ½ grapefruit, peeled
- ½ cup pineapple chunks
- ½ cup coconut water

- ½ tablespoon chia seeds
- ½ cup ice cubes

Instructions:
Blend orange, grapefruit, pineapple, coconut water, chia seeds, and ice cubes until you get a zesty and hydrating morning blend.

Avocado Banana Bliss

Ingredients:
- ½ avocado, peeled and pitted
- ½ banana, frozen
- ½ cup spinach
- ½ cup coconut milk
- ½ tablespoon hemp seeds
- ½ cup water or almond milk

Instructions:
Blend avocado, frozen banana, spinach, coconut milk, hemp seeds, and water or almond milk for a creamy and nutritious breakfast treat.

Chocolate Almond Joy

Ingredients:
- ½ banana, frozen

- ½ tablespoon cocoa powder
- ½ cup almond milk
- ½ tablespoon almond butter
- ½ tablespoon shredded coconut
- ½ teaspoon vanilla extract

Instructions:

Blend frozen banana, cocoa powder, almond milk, almond butter, shredded coconut, and vanilla extract for a guilt-free chocolatey delight.

Blueberry Muffin Smoothie

Ingredients:
- ½ cup blueberries
- ½ cup oats
- ½ cup vanilla Greek yogurt
- ½ cup milk (dairy or plant-based)
- ½ tablespoon honey
- ½ teaspoon cinnamon

Instructions:

Blend blueberries, oats, vanilla Greek yogurt, milk, honey, and cinnamon to capture the essence of a blueberry muffin in a nutritious smoothie.

Spinach Pineapple Paradise

Ingredients:
- ½ cup spinach
- ½ cup pineapple chunks
- ½ banana, frozen
- ½ cup coconut water
- ½ tablespoon chia seeds
- ½ cup ice cubes

Instructions:
Blend spinach, pineapple, frozen banana, coconut water, chia seeds, and ice cubes for a refreshing tropical paradise in a glass.

Mango Coconut Dream

Ingredients:
- ½ cup mango, diced
- ½ cup coconut milk
- ½ cup plain yogurt
- ½ tablespoon shredded coconut
- ½ tablespoon honey
- ½ cup ice cubes

Instructions:

Blend mango, coconut milk, plain yogurt, shredded coconut, honey, and ice cubes for a dreamy and exotic morning concoction.

Peachy Keen Quencher

Ingredients:
- ½ cup peaches, sliced
- ½ cup raspberries
- ½ cup almond milk
- ½ cup plain yogurt
- ½ tablespoon chia seeds
- ½ teaspoon vanilla extract

Instructions:
Blend peaches, raspberries, almond milk, plain yogurt, chia seeds, and vanilla extract for a peachy and satisfying morning quencher.

Protein-Packed Green Machine

Ingredients:
- ½ cup kale, stems removed
- ½ cup cucumber, peeled
- ½ cup green grapes
- ½ cup plain Greek yogurt
- ½ tablespoon hemp seeds

- ½ cup water or coconut water

Instructions:
Blend kale, cucumber, green grapes, Greek yogurt, hemp seeds, and water or coconut water for a protein-packed green smoothie.

Almond Cherry Burst

Ingredients:
- ½ cup cherries, pitted
- ½ cup almond milk
- ½ cup vanilla Greek yogurt
- ½ tablespoon almond butter
- ½ tablespoon honey
- ½ cup ice cubes

Instructions:
Blend cherries, almond milk, vanilla Greek yogurt, almond butter, honey, and ice cubes for a burst of almond-cherry goodness.

Raspberry Lemon Refresher

Ingredients:
- ½ cup raspberries
- ½ lemon, peeled and segmented

- ½ cup coconut water
- ½ cup plain yogurt
- ½ tablespoon chia seeds
- ½ cup ice cubes

Instructions:

Blend raspberries, lemon segments, coconut water, plain yogurt, chia seeds, and ice cubes for a zesty and hydrating morning refresher.

Vanilla Peach Perfection

Ingredients:
- ½ cup peaches, sliced
- ½ teaspoon vanilla extract
- ½ cup almond milk
- ½ cup plain Greek yogurt
- ½ tablespoon honey
- ½ cup ice cubes

Instructions:

Blend peaches, vanilla extract, almond milk, plain Greek yogurt, honey, and ice cubes for a creamy and peachy perfection.

Cranberry Orange Burst

Ingredients:

- ½ cup cranberries (fresh or frozen)
- ½ orange, peeled
- ½ cup vanilla almond milk
- ½ cup plain yogurt
- ½ tablespoon honey
- ½ cup ice cubes

Instructions:

Blend cranberries, orange, vanilla almond milk, plain yogurt, honey, and ice cubes for a burst of cranberry-orange freshness.

Pineapple Coconut Serenity

Ingredients:

- ½ cup pineapple chunks
- ½ cup coconut milk
- ½ cup spinach
- ½ tablespoon chia seeds
- ½ tablespoon shredded coconut
- ½ cup ice cubes

Instructions:

Blend pineapple, coconut milk, spinach, chia seeds, shredded coconut, and ice cubes for a serene and tropical morning treat.

Cinnamon Apple Pie Delight

Ingredients:
- ½ apple, cored and sliced
- ½ teaspoon cinnamon
- ½ cup oats
- ½ cup almond milk
- ½ tablespoon honey
- ½ cup ice cubes

Instructions:
Blend apple slices, cinnamon, oats, almond milk, honey, and ice cubes for a delicious and nutritious apple pie-inspired breakfast delight.

LUNCHTIME ELIXIRS

Veggie Bliss Smoothie

Ingredients:
- ½ cup kale, stems removed
- ½ cucumber, peeled
- ½ celery stalk
- ½ cup carrots, chopped
- ½ green apple, cored
- ½ lemon, juiced
- ½ cup water or coconut water

Instructions:
Blend kale, cucumber, celery, carrots, green apple, lemon juice, and water or coconut water for a refreshing and nutrient-packed veggie elixir.

Protein-Packed Lunch Fix

Ingredients:
- ½ cup spinach
- ½ cup Greek yogurt

- ½ cup pineapple chunks
- ½ banana, frozen
- ½ tablespoon chia seeds
- ½ cup almond milk

Instructions:
Blend spinach, Greek yogurt, pineapple chunks, frozen banana, chia seeds, and almond milk for a protein-rich elixir perfect for a satisfying lunch.

Citrus Zest Refuel

Ingredients:
- ½ orange, peeled
- ½ grapefruit, peeled
- ½ cup strawberries
- ½ cup coconut water
- ½ tablespoon flaxseeds
- ½ cup ice cubes

Instructions:
Blend orange, grapefruit, strawberries, coconut water, flaxseeds, and ice cubes for a zesty and refreshing citrus elixir to refuel your afternoon.

Mediterranean Veggie Boost

Ingredients:
- ½ cup cherry tomatoes
- ½ cucumber, peeled
- ½ bell pepper, any color
- ½ cup olives
- ½ cup feta cheese, crumbled
- ½ cup water or vegetable broth

Instructions:
Blend cherry tomatoes, cucumber, bell pepper, olives, feta cheese, and water or vegetable broth for a savory and satisfying Mediterranean-inspired veggie elixir.

Spicy Tomato Kick

Ingredients:
- ½ cup cherry tomatoes
- ½ cup cucumber, peeled
- ½ celery stalk
- ½ jalapeño, seeds removed
- ½ cup tomato juice
- ½ teaspoon hot sauce

Instructions:

Blend cherry tomatoes, cucumber, celery, jalapeño, tomato juice, and hot sauce for a spicy and invigorating tomato elixir with a kick.

Quinoa Power Blend

Ingredients:
- ½ cup cooked quinoa, cooled
- ½ cup spinach
- ½ avocado, peeled and pitted
- ½ cup plain Greek yogurt
- ½ cup water or almond milk
- ½ tablespoon honey

Instructions:
Blend cooked quinoa, spinach, avocado, Greek yogurt, water or almond milk, and honey for a protein-packed and energizing quinoa elixir.

Green Goddess Elixir

Ingredients:
- ½ cup kale, stems removed
- ½ cucumber, peeled
- ½ avocado, peeled and pitted
- ½ lime, juiced

- ½ tablespoon hemp seeds
- ½ cup coconut water

Instructions:
Blend kale, cucumber, avocado, lime juice, hemp seeds, and coconut water for a Green Goddess elixir that's rich in nutrients and refreshing to the palate.

Sweet Potato Sunshine Elixir

Ingredients:
- ½ cup cooked sweet potato, cooled
- ½ carrot, chopped
- ½ orange, peeled
- ½ cup plain yogurt
- ½ tablespoon turmeric
- ½ cup water or orange juice

Instructions:
Blend cooked sweet potato, carrot, orange, yogurt, turmeric, and water or orange juice for a vibrant and immune-boosting elixir.

Broccoli Bliss Elixir

Ingredients:

- ½ cup broccoli florets
- ½ cucumber, peeled
- ½ green apple, cored
- ½ lemon, juiced
- ½ cup water or vegetable broth
- ½ teaspoon ginger, grated

Instructions:

Blend broccoli, cucumber, green apple, lemon juice, water or vegetable broth, and grated ginger for a nutrient-packed broccoli elixir.

Black Bean Fiesta Elixir

Ingredients:
- ½ cup black beans, cooked and cooled
- ½ cup tomatoes, diced
- ½ avocado, peeled and pitted
- ½ cup cilantro leaves
- ½ lime, juiced
- ½ cup vegetable broth

Instructions:

Blend black beans, tomatoes, avocado, cilantro leaves, lime juice, and vegetable broth for a fiesta-inspired black bean elixir.

Pomegranate Passion Elixir

Ingredients:
- ½ cup pomegranate seeds
- ½ cup raspberries
- ½ cup plain yogurt
- ½ cup coconut water
- ½ tablespoon honey
- ½ cup ice cubes

Instructions:
Blend pomegranate seeds, raspberries, yogurt, coconut water, honey, and ice cubes for a sweet and tangy pomegranate elixir.

Spinach Artichoke Elixir

Ingredients:
- ½ cup spinach
- ½ cup artichoke hearts, canned or cooked
- ½ cup plain Greek yogurt
- ½ lemon, juiced
- ½ teaspoon garlic, minced
- ½ cup vegetable broth

Instructions:

Blend spinach, artichoke hearts, Greek yogurt, lemon juice, minced garlic, and vegetable broth for a savory and satisfying elixir.

Mango Turmeric Elixir

Ingredients:
- ½ cup mango, diced
- ½ teaspoon turmeric
- ½ cup plain yogurt
- ½ cup coconut water
- ½ tablespoon chia seeds
- ½ cup ice cubes

Instructions:
Blend mango, turmeric, yogurt, coconut water, chia seeds, and ice cubes for a tropical and anti-inflammatory mango turmeric elixir.

Cauliflower Cream Elixir

Ingredients:
- ½ cup cauliflower florets, cooked and cooled
- ½ cup cucumber, peeled
- ½ cup coconut milk
- ½ teaspoon cumin

- ½ teaspoon coriander
- ½ cup vegetable broth

Instructions:

Blend cauliflower, cucumber, coconut milk, cumin, coriander, and vegetable broth for a creamy and flavorful cauliflower elixir.

Raspberry Basil Bliss Elixir

Ingredients:
- ½ cup raspberries
- ½ cup cucumber, peeled
- ½ lime, juiced
- ½ cup fresh basil leaves
- ½ tablespoon honey
- ½ cup coconut water

Instructions:

Blend raspberries, cucumber, lime juice, fresh basil leaves, honey, and coconut water for a refreshing and aromatic raspberry basil elixir.

Chickpea Spinach Spectacle

Ingredients:
- ½ cup chickpeas, cooked and cooled

- ½ cup spinach
- ½ cucumber, peeled
- ½ lemon, juiced
- ½ teaspoon cumin
- ½ cup vegetable broth

Instructions:
Blend chickpeas, spinach, cucumber, lemon juice, cumin, and vegetable broth for a protein-packed and nutritious chickpea elixir.

Cilantro Lime Revitalizer

Ingredients:
- ½ cup cilantro leaves
- ½ cucumber, peeled
- ½ lime, juiced
- ½ cup green apple, cored
- ½ cup coconut water
- ½ tablespoon chia seeds

Instructions:
Blend cilantro leaves, cucumber, lime juice, green apple, coconut water, and chia seeds for a revitalizing cilantro lime elixir.

Sweet Potato Spice Elixir

Ingredients:

- ½ cup cooked sweet potato, cooled
- ½ teaspoon cinnamon
- ½ cup plain yogurt
- ½ cup almond milk
- ½ tablespoon maple syrup
- ½ cup ice cubes

Instructions:

Blend cooked sweet potato, cinnamon, yogurt, almond milk, maple syrup, and ice cubes for a warm and comforting sweet potato spice elixir.

Asparagus Avocado Elixir

Ingredients:

- ½ cup asparagus, cooked and cooled
- ½ avocado, peeled and pitted
- ½ cup spinach
- ½ lemon, juiced
- ½ cup vegetable broth
- ½ teaspoon dill

Instructions:

Blend asparagus, avocado, spinach, lemon juice, vegetable broth, and dill for a green and nutrient-packed asparagus avocado elixir.

Blueberry Basil Breeze

Ingredients:
- ½ cup blueberries
- ½ cup cucumber, peeled
- ½ cup fresh basil leaves
- ½ lime, juiced
- ½ tablespoon honey
- ½ cup coconut water

Instructions:
Blend blueberries, cucumber, fresh basil leaves, lime juice, honey, and coconut water for a delightful and aromatic blueberry basil elixir.

SNACK ATTACK

Nutty Banana Bites

Ingredients:
- ½ banana, sliced
- ½ tablespoon almond butter
- ½ tablespoon honey
- ½ tablespoon chia seeds

Instructions:
Spread almond butter on banana slices, drizzle with honey, and sprinkle chia seeds for a quick and satisfying nutty snack.

Greek Yogurt Parfait

Ingredients:
- ½ cup Greek yogurt
- ½ cup mixed berries
- ½ tablespoon granola
- ½ tablespoon honey

Instructions:
Layer Greek yogurt, mixed berries, granola, and drizzle with honey for a delightful and protein-packed parfait.

Apple Cinnamon Crunch

Ingredients:
- ½ apple, sliced
- ½ tablespoon almond butter
- ½ tablespoon granola
- ½ teaspoon cinnamon

Instructions:
Spread almond butter on apple slices, sprinkle with granola, and dust with cinnamon for a crunchy and sweet snack.

Veggie Sticks with Hummus

Ingredients:
- ½ cup carrot and cucumber sticks
- ½ cup hummus for dipping

Instructions:
Pair carrot and cucumber sticks with hummus for a refreshing and crunchy veggie snack.

Trail Mix Medley

Ingredients:

- ½ cup mixed nuts (almonds, walnuts, cashews)
- ½ cup dried fruit (raisins, cranberries)
- ½ cup dark chocolate chips

Instructions:
Combine mixed nuts, dried fruit, and dark chocolate chips for a flavorful and energy-boosting trail mix.

Rice Cake Delight

Ingredients:
- ½ rice cake
- ½ tablespoon almond butter
- ½ banana, sliced
- ½ tablespoon honey

Instructions:
Spread almond butter on a rice cake, top with banana slices, and drizzle with honey for a crunchy and satisfying treat.

Caprese Skewers

Ingredients:
- ½ cup cherry tomatoes

- • ½ mozzarella cheese, cubed
- • ½ tablespoon balsamic glaze

Instructions:
Thread cherry tomatoes and mozzarella cubes onto skewers, drizzle with balsamic glaze for a refreshing Caprese snack.

Cottage Cheese Crunch

Ingredients:
- • ½ cup cottage cheese
- • ½ cup pineapple chunks
- • ½ tablespoon sunflower seeds

Instructions:
Mix cottage cheese with pineapple chunks and sprinkle with sunflower seeds for a protein-packed and crunchy snack.

Edamame Explosion

Ingredients:
- • ½ cup edamame, steamed
- • ½ teaspoon sea salt

Instructions:

Sprinkle steamed edamame with sea salt for a simple and nutritious salty snack.

Avocado Toast Bites

Ingredients:
- ½ slice whole-grain toast
- ½ avocado, mashed
- Sprinkle of red pepper flakes
- ½ teaspoon lemon juice

Instructions:
Spread mashed avocado on toast, sprinkle with red pepper flakes, and drizzle with lemon juice for a tasty avocado toast bite.

Almond Joy Energy Balls

Ingredients:
- ½ cup almonds
- ¼ cup dates, pitted
- ½ cup shredded coconut
- ½ tablespoon cocoa powder

Instructions:

Blend almonds, dates, shredded coconut, and cocoa powder. Form into balls for a sweet and energy-packed snack.

Stuffed Bell Pepper Halves

Ingredients:
- ½ bell pepper, sliced
- ½ cup hummus
- ½ cup cherry tomatoes, halved

Instructions:
Fill bell pepper halves with hummus and top with cherry tomatoes for a colorful and satisfying snack.

Popcorn Fiesta

Ingredients:
- ½ cup air-popped popcorn
- ½ teaspoon chili powder
- ½ teaspoon nutritional yeast

Instructions:
Sprinkle air-popped popcorn with chili powder and nutritional yeast for a flavorful and guilt-free popcorn fiesta.

Guacamole and Veggie Dippers

Ingredients:
- ½ avocado, mashed
- ½ tablespoon lime juice
- ½ cup bell pepper strips and cucumber slices for dipping

Instructions:
Mix mashed avocado with lime juice and serve with bell pepper strips and cucumber slices for a refreshing guacamole snack.

Spinach and Feta Stuffed Mushrooms

Ingredients:
- ½ cup mushrooms, cleaned and stems removed
- ½ cup spinach, chopped
- ½ tablespoon feta cheese, crumbled

Instructions:
Stuff mushrooms with chopped spinach and crumbled feta, then bake for a savory and nutritious snack.

Peanut Butter Banana Quesadilla

Ingredients:
- ½ whole-grain tortilla
- ½ tablespoon peanut butter
- ½ banana, sliced

Instructions:
Spread peanut butter on a tortilla, top with banana slices, fold, and toast for a delicious quesadilla.

Tuna Cucumber Cups

Ingredients:
- ½ cucumber, sliced into rounds
- ½ cup tuna salad (canned tuna, mayo, celery)
- ½ cherry tomatoes, halved

Instructions:
Fill cucumber rounds with tuna salad and top with cherry tomato halves for a light and protein-packed snack.

Berry Yogurt Bark

Ingredients:
- ½ cup Greek yogurt
- ½ cup mixed berries
- ½ tablespoon honey

Instructions:
Mix Greek yogurt with mixed berries, spread on a baking sheet, and drizzle with honey. Freeze, then break into pieces for a cool and fruity yogurt bark.

Hummus Stuffed Mini Peppers

Ingredients:
- ½ cup mini bell peppers, halved
- ½ cup hummus
- ½ teaspoon paprika

Instructions:
Fill mini bell pepper halves with hummus and sprinkle with paprika for a tasty and colorful snack.

Dark Chocolate Dipped Strawberries

Ingredients:
- ½ cup strawberries, washed and dried

- ½ ounce dark chocolate, melted

Instructions:
Dip strawberries in melted dark chocolate and let them cool for a sweet and indulgent snack.

DINNER IN A GLASS

Garden Fresh Delight
- ½ cup cherry tomatoes
- ½ cucumber, peeled
- ¼ cup red bell pepper
- ¼ cup feta cheese
- 1 tablespoon olive oil
- 1 teaspoon balsamic vinegar
- Salt and pepper to taste

Protein Powerhouse
- ½ cup cooked quinoa
- ½ cup black beans, cooked
- ¼ cup corn kernels
- ½ avocado, diced
- 2 tablespoons salsa
- Fresh cilantro for garnish

Creamy Avocado Basil Blend
- ½ avocado
- 1 cup spinach
- ¼ cup fresh basil leaves
- 1 tablespoon pine nuts
- 2 tablespoons Greek yogurt
- Lemon juice for brightness

Thai Coconut Curry Elixir

- ½ cup cooked rice noodles
- ½ cup coconut milk
- 1 tablespoon red curry paste
- ½ cup cooked chicken, shredded
- Bean sprouts for crunch
- Fresh cilantro for garnish

Mediterranean Chickpea Magic

- ½ cup cooked chickpeas
- ½ cup cherry tomatoes, halved
- ¼ cup Kalamata olives, sliced
- 2 tablespoons feta cheese
- 1 tablespoon olive oil
- Fresh oregano for garnish

Pesto Primavera Elegance

- ½ cup cooked spiralized zucchini
- ¼ cup cherry tomatoes
- 2 tablespoons pesto sauce
- 1 tablespoon pine nuts
- Parmesan shavings for topping

Spicy Black Bean Fiesta

- ½ cup black beans, cooked
- ¼ cup corn kernels
- ¼ cup diced red onion

- ½ jalapeño, seeds removed
- 2 tablespoons salsa verde
- Fresh cilantro for garnish

Teriyaki Tofu Temptation
- ½ cup baked tofu, cubed
- ½ cup broccoli florets, steamed
- ¼ cup carrots, julienned
- 2 tablespoons teriyaki sauce
- Sesame seeds for garnish

Caesar Salad Sip
- ½ cup chopped Romaine lettuce
- ¼ cup cherry tomatoes
- 2 tablespoons Caesar dressing
- 1 tablespoon grated Parmesan cheese
- Croutons for crunch

Smoky Lentil Salsa Surprise
- ½ cup cooked lentils
- ¼ cup diced tomatoes
- 2 tablespoons salsa
- 1 tablespoon chopped red onion
- Smoked paprika for flavor

Caprese Capriccio
- ½ cup cherry tomatoes, halved

- ½ cup fresh mozzarella balls
- ¼ cup basil leaves
- Balsamic glaze for drizzling
- Salt and pepper to taste

Sweet Potato & Chickpea Harmony

- ½ cup roasted sweet potato cubes
- ½ cup cooked chickpeas
- 2 tablespoons tahini
- Lemon juice for brightness
- Cumin for flavor

Greek Gyro Glass

- ½ cup cooked quinoa
- ½ cup cucumber, diced
- ¼ cup cherry tomatoes, halved
- ¼ cup red onion, sliced
- Tzatziki sauce for drizzling
- Fresh dill for garnish

Broccoli Cheddar Bliss

- ½ cup steamed broccoli
- ½ cup cheddar cheese, shredded
- 2 tablespoons plain yogurt
- 1 clove garlic, minced
- Nutmeg for a hint of warmth

Southwest Fiesta Fling

- ½ cup black beans, cooked
- ¼ cup corn kernels
- ¼ cup diced red bell pepper
- ½ avocado, diced
- 2 tablespoons salsa
- Fresh cilantro for garnish

Citrus Shrimp Spectacle

- ½ cup cooked shrimp, peeled
- ½ orange, peeled and segmented
- ¼ cup cucumber, diced
- 1 tablespoon lime juice
- Avocado slices for richness

Quinoa Caesar Cascade

- ½ cup cooked quinoa
- ½ cup chopped Romaine lettuce
- 2 tablespoons Caesar dressing
- 1 tablespoon grated Parmesan cheese
- Croutons for crunch

Roasted Red Pepper Euphoria

- ½ cup roasted red peppers
- ½ cup cherry tomatoes
- ¼ cup feta cheese
- 2 tablespoons olive oil

- Fresh basil for garnish

Avocado Ranch Revelry
- ½ avocado
- 2 tablespoons Greek yogurt
- ¼ cup diced tomatoes
- ¼ cup diced cucumber
- Ranch dressing for drizzling

Spiced Lentil Pumpkin Pleasure
- ½ cup cooked lentils
- ½ cup pumpkin puree
- 1 tablespoon curry powder
- 2 tablespoons coconut milk
- Cilantro for garnish

For each recipe, blend the ingredients until smooth, adjust seasoning to taste, and enjoy your unique "Dinner in a Glass" experience!

POST-WORKOUT POWER BLENDS:

Muscle Recovery Blend
- ½ cup Greek yogurt
- ½ banana
- 1 scoop whey protein powder
- 1 tablespoon almond butter
- 1 cup water or milk of choice

Hydration Replenisher
- ½ cup coconut water
- -½ cup watermelon chunks
- 1 tablespoon chia seeds
- 1 teaspoon honey
- Ice cubes for refreshing coolness

Superfood Refuel
- ½ cup kale
- ½ cup blueberries
- 1 tablespoon hemp seeds
- 1 tablespoon flaxseeds
- 1 cup almond milk

Nutty Chocolate Bliss

- ½ cup chocolate milk (or chocolate almond milk)
- ½ banana
- 1 tablespoon peanut butter
- 1 scoop chocolate protein powder
- Ice cubes for thickness

Green Power Protein Punch
- ½ cup spinach
- ½ cup pineapple chunks
- 1 scoop plant-based protein powder
- 1 tablespoon chia seeds
- 1 cup coconut water

Berry Blast Recovery
- ½ cup mixed berries (strawberries, blueberries and raspberries)
- ½ cup cottage cheese
- 1 tablespoon honey
- 1 cup water or milk of choice

Tropical Turmeric Refuel
- ½ cup mango chunks
- ½ banana
- 1 teaspoon turmeric
- 1 tablespoon Greek yogurt
- 1 cup coconut water

Almond Joy Rejuvenator

- ½ cup almond milk
- ½ cup coconut milk
- 1 tablespoon almond butter
- 1 tablespoon cocoa powder
- Ice cubes for thickness

Quinoa Power Protein

- ½ cup cooked quinoa
- ½ cup strawberries
- 1 scoop vanilla protein powder
- 1 tablespoon almond milk
- Ice cubes for refreshing coolness

Avocado Banana Elixir

- ½ avocado
- ½ banana
- 1 tablespoon chia seeds
- 1 tablespoon honey
- 1 cup almond milk

These post-workout power recipes are designed to support muscle recovery, replenish hydration, and refuel your body with essential nutrients. Adjust ingredients to fit your preferences and dietary needs. Enjoy!

5-minute magic smoothie hacks and time-saving tips for busy lifestyles:

Flash Freeze Cubes:
- Blend favorite smoothie ingredients (fruits, yogurt, greens).
- Pour the mixture into ice cube trays and freeze.
- When ready to make a quick smoothie, pop a few cubes into the blender, add liquid, and blend.

Pre-Packaged Smoothie Bags:
- Prepare individual smoothie ingredient bags during meal prep.
- Combine fruits, greens, and any dry ingredients.
- Store in the freezer, then grab a bag, add liquid, and blend for a speedy smoothie.

Overnight Oats Fusion:
- Mix rolled oats, yogurt, and liquid in a jar.
- Refrigerate overnight.

- In the morning, blend the overnight oats with fruits for a nutritious and quick breakfast smoothie.

Protein Power Packs:
- Pre-measure protein powder, seeds, and nuts into small containers.
- Keep these "power packs" handy for a quick protein boost in any smoothie.

Citrus Zest Boost:
- Keep citrus zest (lemon, lime, or orange) in the freezer.
- Add a pinch to your smoothie for a burst of flavor without the prep time of peeling.

These 5-minute magic smoothie hacks and time-saving tips are perfect for those hectic days. Enjoy your quick and nutritious smoothies without compromising on taste or nutrition!

7-Day Smoothie Challenge: Elevate Your Daily Nutrition!

Embark on a week-long journey to boost your well-being with the 7-Day Smoothie Challenge. Here's how:

1. Daily Nutrient Boost: Enjoy a different smoothie each day, packed with a variety of fruits, veggies, and superfoods. Challenge yourself to explore new flavors and discover the diverse health benefits of each ingredient.

2. Share Your Journey: Connect with fellow participants by sharing your daily smoothie creations on social media. Use the hashtag #SmoothieBoostChallenge to inspire and be inspired. Share recipes, tips, and the joy of a daily nutrient-packed treat.

3. Experiment and Customize: Tailor your smoothies to your taste and health goals. Whether you're focusing on energy, immunity, or detox, use this challenge to find the perfect blend that suits your lifestyle.

4. Nutrition Reinforcement: Reinforce the importance of daily nutrition as a foundation for overall well-being. Use this challenge as a springboard to establish a habit of incorporating healthy, delicious smoothies into your routine.

Day 1: Tropical Kickstart

- ½ cup pineapple chunks
- ½ banana
- 1 cup coconut water
- 1 tablespoon chia seeds

Blend and enjoy this refreshing tropical blend to kickstart your challenge.

Day 2: Berry Bliss Burst

- ½ cup mixed berries (strawberries, blueberries and raspberries)
- ½ cup Greek yogurt
- 1 tablespoon honey
- 1 cup almond milk

Blend for a burst of antioxidants and creamy goodness.

Day 3: Green Energy Elixir

- ½ cup spinach
- ½ cucumber
- ½ green apple
- 1 tablespoon flaxseeds
- 1 cup water

Power up with this nutrient-packed green elixir.

Day 4: Citrus Zest Refresher

- ½ orange (peeled)
- ½ grapefruit (peeled)
- 1 tablespoon Greek yogurt
- 1 tablespoon hemp seeds
- 1 cup water

Refresh your senses with the zesty goodness of citrus.

Day 5: Chocolate Banana Delight

- ½ banana
- 1 tablespoon cocoa powder
- 1 tablespoon almond butter
- 1 scoop chocolate protein powder
- 1 cup almond milk

Satisfy your sweet cravings with this chocolaty treat.

Day 6: Berry Green Fusion

- ½ cup kale
- ½ cup mixed berries (strawberries, blueberries and raspberries)
- 1 tablespoon chia seeds
- 1 cup coconut water

Fuse the goodness of greens and berries for a vibrant mix.

Day 7: Creamy Avocado Dream

- ½ avocado
- ½ banana
- 1 tablespoon coconut flakes

- 1 tablespoon honey
- 1 cup almond milk

Wrap up your challenge with this creamy and nourishing avocado dream.

Remember to share your creations on social media using #SmoothieChallenge. Enjoy this week of delicious and nutritious smoothies!

Monthly Transformation Tracker: Your Personal Growth Compass!

Kickstart a transformative journey with the Monthly Transformation Tracker. Here's how to make the most of it:

1. Goal Setting: At the beginning of each month, set specific health and wellness goals. Whether it's increasing daily steps, hydrating more, or trying new fitness routines, define clear objectives.

2. Progress Monitoring: Regularly track your progress throughout the month. Utilize a combination of methods, such as journaling, taking photos, and using fitness metrics, to gauge your achievements and identify areas for improvement.

3. Reflect and Adjust: Take time at the end of each month to reflect on your experiences. Celebrate victories, learn from challenges, and adjust your goals for the upcoming month. This reflective practice creates a positive cycle of self-improvement.

4. Consistency is Key: Embrace the idea that transformation is a gradual process. Consistency in tracking and adjusting your goals will lead to sustainable and positive changes over time.

By combining the 7-Day Smoothie Challenge and the Monthly Transformation Tracker, you'll create a holistic approach to nurturing your well-being. These tools are designed to be accessible, flexible, and supportive, empowering you to make tangible and lasting improvements in your health and lifestyle. Cheers to your transformative journey!

Conclusion: Your Journey to a Healthier You

As you conclude this transformative journey, reflect on the steps you've taken toward a healthier and more vibrant life. Your commitment to the 7-Day Smoothie Challenge and the Monthly Transformation Tracker has laid the foundation for positive change. Here's a brief recap and encouragement for the road ahead:

1. Discovering Nutrient-Packed Joy:
- Throughout the 7-Day Smoothie Challenge, you explored a spectrum of flavors and experienced the joy of nutrient-packed smoothies. Celebrate the newfound appreciation for wholesome ingredients and the positive impact on your well-being.

2. Tracking Progress and Growth:
- The Monthly Transformation Tracker became your compass for personal growth. By setting clear goals, consistently monitoring progress, and

embracing a reflective mindset, you've cultivated a habit of self-improvement.

3. Celebrating Small Wins:

- Acknowledge and celebrate every small victory. Whether it's completing a challenging workout, consistently meeting your hydration goals, or trying a new ingredient, each accomplishment contributes to your overall success.

4. Building Lasting Habits:

- Transformation is a journey, not a destination. Use the habits formed during this challenge as building blocks for a sustainable, healthier lifestyle. Small, consistent changes compound over time, leading to profound and lasting results.

5. Continuing the Momentum:

- Your journey doesn't end here—it evolves. Continue to explore, experiment, and refine your approach to health and wellness. Embrace the journey, adapt to new challenges, and stay committed to the positive changes you've initiated.

Remember, this is just the beginning. Your commitment to a healthier you is a continuous, evolving process. Embrace the lessons learned, maintain the positive habits, and let them guide you toward a future filled with well-being and vitality. Your journey to a healthier you is ongoing—keep moving forward with determination and optimism. Cheers to your continued success!

THANK YOU

Dear Readers,

As we wrap up this incredible journey towards better health, we want to extend our heartfelt gratitude to you. Your commitment to exploring nutritious recipes, embracing transformative challenges, and prioritizing your well-being has been truly inspiring.

In every smoothie blended, challenge accepted, and healthy choice made, you've contributed to a community dedicated to fostering positive change. Your enthusiasm and engagement have made this journey richer and more meaningful.

Thank you for being an essential part of our health-focused community. We appreciate your trust, commitment, and the shared passion for a healthier, more vibrant life. As we continue to explore new recipes, challenges, and wellness tips, we look forward to supporting each other on this ongoing journey towards optimal well-being.

With gratitude,

AURORA HENDRIX

9 798876 731197